REVIEW OF THE ISSUES RELATED TO THE PREVENTION, DETECTION, AND ERADICATION OF AVIAN INFLUENZA

HEARING

BEFORE THE

COMMITTEE ON AGRICULTURE
HOUSE OF REPRESENTATIVES

ONE HUNDRED NINTH CONGRESS

FIRST SESSION

NOVEMBER 16, 2005

Serial No. 109–21

Printed for the use of the Committee on Agriculture
www.agriculture.house.gov

U.S. GOVERNMENT PRINTING OFFICE

25–313 PDF   WASHINGTON : 2006

For sale by the Superintendent of Documents, U.S. Government Printing Office
Internet: bookstore.gpo.gov   Phone: toll free (866) 512–1800; DC area (202) 512–1800
Fax: (202) 512–2250   Mail: Stop SSOP, Washington, DC 20402–0001

COMMITTEE ON AGRICULTURE

BOB GOODLATTE, Virginia, *Chairman*

JOHN A. BOEHNER, Ohio,
   Vice Chairman
RICHARD W. POMBO, California
TERRY EVERETT, Alabama
FRANK D. LUCAS, Oklahoma
JERRY MORAN, Kansas
WILLIAM L. JENKINS, Tennessee
GIL GUTKNECHT, Minnesota
ROBIN HAYES, North Carolina
TIMOTHY V. JOHNSON, Illinois
TOM OSBORNE, Nebraska
MIKE PENCE, Indiana
SAM GRAVES, Missouri
JO BONNER, Alabama
MIKE ROGERS, Alabama
STEVE KING, Iowa
MARILYN N. MUSGRAVE, Colorado
RANDY NEUGEBAUER, Texas
CHARLES W. BOUSTANY, JR., LOUISIANA
JOHN J.H. "JOE" SCHWARZ, Michigan
JOHN R. "RANDY" KUHL, JR., New York
VIRGINIA FOXX, North Carolina
K. MICHAEL CONAWAY, Texas
JEFF FORTENBERRY, Nebraska
JEAN SCHMIDT, Ohio

COLLIN C. PETERSON, Minnesota,
   Ranking Minority Member
TIM HOLDEN, Pennsylvania
MIKE McINTYRE, North Carolina
BOB ETHERIDGE, North Carolina
JOE BACA, California
ED CASE, Hawaii
DENNIS A. CARDOZA, California
DAVID SCOTT, Georgia
JIM MARSHALL, Georgia
STEPHANIE HERSETH, South Dakota
G.K. BUTTERFIELD, North Carolina
HENRY CUELLAR, Texas
CHARLIE MELANCON, Louisiana
JIM COSTA, California
JOHN T. SALAZAR, Colorado
JOHN BARROW, Georgia
EARL POMEROY, North Dakota
LEONARD L. BOSWELL, Iowa
RICK LARSEN, Washington
LINCOLN DAVIS, Tennessee
BEN CHANDLER, Kentucky

PROFESSIONAL STAFF

WILLIAM E. O'CONNER, JR., *Staff Director*
KEVIN J. KRAMP, *Chief Counsel*
JOHN HAUGEN, *Communications Director*
ROBERT L. LAREW, *Minority Staff Director*

(II)

CONTENTS

REVIEW OF THE ISSUES RELATED TO THE PREVENTION, DETECTION, AND ERADICATION OF AVIAN INFLUENZA

WEDNESDAY, NOVEMBER 16, 2005

HOUSE OF REPRESENTATIVES,
COMMITTEE ON AGRICULTURE,
Washington, DC.

The committee met, pursuant to call, at 10 a.m., in room 1300, Longworth House Office Building, Hon. Bob Goodlatte (chairman of the committee) presiding.

Present: Representatives Moran, Gutknecht, Hayes, Johnson, Musgrave, Foxx, Conaway, Schmidt, Peterson, Holden, Etheridge, Baca, Herseth, Butterfield, Cuellar, Costa, Salazar, Pomeroy, Larsen, Davis and Chandler.

Staff present: Pete Thomson, John Goldberg, Pamilyn Miller, Elizabeth Parker, Tyler Wegmeyer, Callista Gingrich, clerk; Lindsey Correa, and Chandler Goule.

OPENING STATEMENT OF HON. BOB GOODLATTE, A REPRESENTATIVE IN CONGRESS FROM THE COMMONWEALTH OF VIRGINIA

The CHAIRMAN. Good morning. This hearing of the House Committee on Agriculture to review the issues related to the prevention, detection and eradication of avian influenza will come to order.

As I know Dr. DeHaven has been quite busy lately, I would like to thank him for taking the time to testify before the House Agriculture Committee regarding avian influenza. I know you have been traveling to Southeast Asia and recently returned from Geneva where you participated in a meeting of the United Nations World Health Organization on the topic of avian influenza.

Recently the agenda of media and Governments worldwide have been consumed by discussions regarding protection, detection and eradication of AI. These conversations have not been without consequences. A recent estimate suggests disruptions in poultry consumption associated with avian influenza are costing the U.S. poultry industry some $88 million per month.

Members of Congress and many constituents I have spoken with are struggling to sort facts from conjecture, and animal health issues from human health issues. I thought it would be helpful for the committee to get a clear understanding of what is known, what is unknown, and what is being done about the portion of the issue we have direct jurisdiction over, avian influenza in poultry.

My own experience with poultry producers is that concern about avian influenza predates the current attention to the issue. It is my understanding that low pathogenic avian influenza has been observed for nearly 100 years. Consequently, producers and processors have developed strategies for managing this problem and continually invest considerable time and resources to prevent introduction of AI into their flocks. With the agriculture community, AI is a well-understood challenge that is already a part of their production routine.

As I alluded to earlier, there are at least two major dimensions to the avian influenza discussion, human health and, the subject of today's hearing, animal health; however, there are other elements as well. For instance, several aspects of the President's avian influenza funding request, issues associated with wild migratory foul and live bird markets, the role of traditional production practices in other nations, the economics of consumption changes, and the impact of international exotic bird trade, to name a few, have a place in the avian flu discussion.

While these issues will be briefly touched on today, we may have a need to have additional hearings to examine these issues in greater detail. Today's hearing will give us a common foundation to guide our thinking on this important issue, and I look forward to Dr. DeHaven's testimony and the questions of my colleagues.

So at this time we are very pleased to welcome our witness, Dr. Ron DeHaven, who is the Administrator of the Animal and Plant Health Inspection Service of the U.S. Department of Agriculture.

Dr. DeHaven, welcome back to the committee.

STATEMENT OF W. RON DeHAVEN, ADMINISTRATOR, ANIMAL AND PLANT HEALTH INSPECTION SERVICE, U.S. DEPARTMENT OF AGRICULTURE,

Dr. DeHAVEN. Thank you.

Mr. Chairman and members of the committee, thank you for the opportunity to testify regarding the Department of Agriculture's extensive efforts to protect U.S. poultry from avian influenza.

In recent months, a highly pathogenic strain of H5N1 avian influenza virus has been spreading across poultry populations in several Southeast Asian and Eastern European countries. There have also been documented cases of the virus affecting humans who have been in direct contact with sick birds. There is worldwide concern that this H5N1 virus might mutate, cross the species barrier, and touch off a human influenza pandemic.

With this in mind, USDA's poultry health safeguarding programs are more important than ever, and we have bolstered our efforts across the board in response to the evolving disease threat overseas.

We also believe it is critical to effectively address the disease in poultry populations in the affected countries. Implementation of effective biosecurity measures, in concert with control and eradication programs, will go a long way towards reducing the amount of virus in these H5N1-affected countries, and thereby minimize the potential for this virus to spread to poultry in other areas of the world. These actions, if effectively implemented, would diminish the potential for a human influenza pandemic as well.

As you mentioned, Mr. Chairman, last week I attended an international meeting on avian influenza, and I can report that there is widespread concern regarding this disease, as well as a strong commitment to work through international organizations to address the disease and improve the animal health infrastructure of countries in the region. That is why it is imperative that the United States remains engaged and shares resources and expertise with the officials in these countries.

Here in the United States, the National Strategy for Pandemic Influenza announced by President Bush on November 1 reflects the importance of these proactive measures on the animal health front. The President requested $91.35 million in emergency funds for USDA to further intensify its surveillance here at home, and to deliver increased assistance to countries impacted by the disease in hopes of preventing further spread of avian influenza.

With that introduction, I want to touch on a few more specific key points that I hope will help frame our discussion this morning. With regard to birds, avian influenza viruses are divided into two groups, low pathogenic avian influenza, or low path AI, and highly pathogenic, or high path AI. The highly pathogenic virus has typically produced far more severe clinical signs and higher mortality in birds than the lower pathogenic avian influenza viruses. Low path AI has been identified in the United States and around the world since the early 1900's. It is relatively common to detect low path, just as human flu viruses are a common finding in people; however, most avian influenza viruses found in birds do not pose any significant health risk to humans.

Highly pathogenic AI has been in found in poultry in the United States three times, in 1924, 1983, and 2004. The 1983 outbreak was the largest, ultimately resulting in the destruction of 17 million birds in Pennsylvania and Virginia before the virus was finally contained and eradicated. In contrast, the 2004 high path incident, it was in a flock of 6,600 birds in Texas. It was quickly found and eradicated. There were no significant human health implications or reports of human health problems in connection with any of these outbreaks.

In domestic poultry, the greatest concern has been infections with the H5 and H7 strains of the virus, which can either be highly pathogenic or low pathogenic. The low pathogenic H5 and H7 viruses are always of concern because they have shown a potential to mutate to the highly pathogenic form of the disease. Given these risks, safeguarding systems against avian influenza are robust and they are encompassing, among other things, trade restrictions on poultry and poultry products from overseas.

We have in place antismuggling programs; aggressive, targeted surveillance in commercial poultry operations and the live bird marketing system in the United States. We have cooperative efforts and information sharing with the States and the industry, and outreach to producers regarding the need for effective on-farm biosecurity measures.

The USDA and our partners, including the Department of Interior, have also been looking for signs of avian influenza in wild birds in the United States, particularly in the Alaska migratory bird flyway, as we know these birds can serve as a reservoir for the disease.

Our ability to respond to a detection of avian influenza is designed to be just as robust as our safeguarding system. For highly pathogenic avian influenza, as well as for the low path strains of H5 and H7, APHIS would work with States to quarantine affected premises, clean and disinfect those premises after the birds had been depopulated and disposed of. Positive highly pathogenic AI flocks would be depopulated, and meat from the affected flocks would not enter the animal food or human food chains. Surveillance testing would also be conducted in a quarantine zone in the surrounding area to ensure that the virus had been completely contained and eradicated.

On the trade front, there is an important new World Organization for Animal Health, or OIE, standard for avian influenza. This new standard obligates member countries to report any positive notifiable avian influenza test result. This notifiable avian influenza would include reporting all highly pathogenic strains of AI, as well as low pathogenic strains of H5 and H7 subtypes detected in commercial poultry flocks. The OIE does not recommend trade restrictions for non-H5 or H7 low pathogenic strains of the virus.

APHIS continues to work with its trading partners to promote the application of this new OIE standard. And in the event of any avian influenza outbreak, we would, of course, work to control and eradicate the disease, and also to demonstrate to trading partners that measures put in place were effective in controlling and eradicating the virus. APHIS would then urge trading partners to regionalize the United States for the disease, effectively allowing trade in poultry and poultry products to continue from unaffected areas.

Even though no human cases of avian influenza have been confirmed from eating properly prepared poultry, I would still like to end by reinforcing a few key food safety messages. These are especially important as we look forward to the Thanksgiving holiday. The proper handling and cooking of poultry provides protection from all manner of viruses and bacteria, including avian influenza. Important safety steps include washing hands, utensils and surfaces that have come in contact with raw poultry, fish and meats with warm soap and water. Avoid cross-contamination of other foods with raw meat, poultry and fish and their juices. And, of course, cook meat thoroughly and use a food thermometer. Cook ground turkey and chicken to a temperature of 165 degrees; chicken and turkey breast to 170 degrees Fahrenheit; and whole birds, legs, thighs and wings to 180 degrees Fahrenheit. Obviously, never consume raw or uncooked poultry or poultry products, and all meat products and other perishables should be refrigerated promptly after serving.

With that, Mr. Chairman, I would end my statement, but I look forward to answering any questions that you may have. Thank you again for the opportunity to testify before the committee on this important topic.

[The prepared statement of Dr. DeHaven appears at the conclusion of the hearing.]

The CHAIRMAN. Thank you, Dr. DeHaven.

In my enthusiasm to get to your testimony, I cut out my partner here Mr. Peterson. So with my apologies, which I hope he will accept, I am going to turn to him for his opening remarks and for his questions to you. The gentleman from Minnesota is recognized.

Mr. PETERSON. Thank you, Mr. Chairman. That is all right, we can shorten up the process a little bit.

I just want to associate myself with your remarks. I think your concerns are similar to mine. Coming from Minnesota, the largest turkey-producing area of the country, and your chickens, and I think you are one of the largest chicken producers, so I think we have similar concerns.

Could you explain to me, Doctor, how this Texas flock acquired this high path, and how that got into that flock, if you know? And also, I am familiar with the low path, but what is the difference between the low path and the high path in terms of the impact on a lower; is there some different way of treating it, or is it more— one more serious than the other?

Dr. DeHAVEN. With regard to the high path avian influenza outbreak in Texas in 2004, we never were able to definitively determine where it came from. However, by looking at the DNA sequencing of the virus, it is very similar to a virus that had been circulating in Mexico and other parts of Central and South America. So we would imagine that it had entered the United States from another country, but again, we were never able to determine that.

I do think, however, that that particular situation points out the fact that we have very good surveillance in place. The fact that we were able to detect that in the index flock before it even had the potential to spread to one other flock is an indication of good surveillance, and, of course, the key to containment and eradication is early detection.

With regard to the difference between a highly pathogenic virus and a low pathogenic virus at the producer level, it really gets down to the clinical signs and the effect on the birds, and the percentage of birds that might die. Even with a low pathogenic avian influenza virus, particularly an H5 or an H7 subtype, there is typically some increase in mortality in the birds, some drop in egg production in layer flocks. On the other hand, if we are talking about a highly pathogenic virus, it can kill 50 percent or more of the birds. The clinical signs are very, very proanounced, and the economic losses just from the virus itself are significant.

So as is the case with this H5N1 virus that is currently circulating in parts of Southeast Asia and Europe, the mortality is high. If there is a positive to that, it is that if there were incursion of that particular virus into the United States, between our testing program and the mortality that we would expect to see, we would quickly be able to identify that virus, and, again, we have the infrastructure and the systems in place to quickly respond.

Mr. PETERSON. Thank you. I agree, I have been in a lot of poultry operations, and I think they have got this under control.

And all this stuff that you read in the media about the migratory birds and so forth, it never was clear to me what part of Canada these birds were in and what they were, if they were geese or ducks, and where they migrate. Do you know all that information?

And in our area, it would be hard to understand how that could have any impact on these commercial operations. I mean, supposedly if some people have a bunch of tamed geese in their pond or something, maybe they could get infected, but these migratory birds, the likelihood of them having any impact on a commercial operation that has got the controls in place would be highly unlikely, wouldn't they?

Dr. DeHaven. Congressman, with regard to the Canadian testing of migratory birds, they were doing testing in a number of provinces, and it is my understanding that the province of Manitoba and one other province had samples that were positive for avian influenza viruses. This is no surprise at all.

Mr. Peterson. Is that low path or high path?

Dr. DeHaven. It was low pathogenic avian influenza viruses. They are still doing the definitive subtyping. They did have some H5 viruses; there may or may not be some H5N1s. But what we do know is there is no evidence that they have the Southeast Asian strain of virus, and, in fact, in talking with the director of their laboratory last week in Geneva at that meeting, he indicated that so far all of their testing has confirmed that these are North American strains of avian influenza viruses, viruses that are endemic in wild migratory bird populations in North America and represent no increased risk from what we historically have had.

With regard to the threat that they pose, clearly I think it would be prudent for us to continue and expand upon the migratory bird surveillance testing that we are doing, and indeed with the additional monies that the President is requesting, we would greatly enhance our surveillance of migratory birds. But that simply provides an early warning system; it helps us to know what viruses are present in those birds and what risks they represent. But as you are alluding to, it is important to note that in commercial production in the United States, the vast majority of our birds are raised indoors, providing some protection from exposure to migratory birds that might be infected.

I would also point out that the biosecurity measures employed by our commercial industry are extensive. Because of outbreaks of low path avian influenza, because of the exotic newcastle disease situation in California, they understand the importance of good biosecurity. And if you start from the premise that every bird out there potentially is carrying a harmful virus, and you employ good biosecurity measures, assuming that any bird could potentially be a risk, then you protect yourself from this Southeast Asian H5N1 virus or any other virus that those birds might be carrying.

Mr. Peterson. If I could just finish, Mr. Chairman. I don't know what kind of public information system you have or what you are doing to try to educate the public. I think there is a lot of misinformation out there. And one of the things with this migratory bird issue, I have had a number of people that hunt ducks and geese ask me whether they should go hunting or not this year. So there is a lack of understanding, I think, because of this publicity about what is going on is not any different than what has always been going on. And have you been trying to do anything to get people to understand that? Or it may be difficult to break through, given all the hysteria that has been stirred up, but——

Dr. DeHAVEN. Congressman Peterson, we have been working diligently because of precisely that concern, the concern that because of all of the media frenzy about the Southeast Asian/European H5N1 virus that we, in fact, tomorrow could find a low path avian influenza virus, something that typically happens two or three or four times a year, and the media and the public would confuse that with this H5N1. So we held a press conference at the Department the week before last primarily for the purpose of educating the media and the public to the fact that there is no evidence to suggest that we have this particular H5N1 virus from Asia in either the human or animal populations in this country.

In terms of getting the word out about biosecurity with our commercial producers as well as individuals that may have back yard flocks, last year we embarked upon a $4 million biosecurity campaign, again stressing the importance of good biosecurity and the threat that is constantly out there. And so just very easy practical measures that anyone from back yard birds to a commercial poultry organization can employ to provide a very good level of protection.

With regard to hunting, and even more specifically with regard to eating poultry with the upcoming Thanksgiving holidays upon us, again, no evidence to suggest that we have any incursion of that H5N1 virus. If it were to come here, we have the infrastructure, the response mechanisms in place to quickly respond and eradicate it. And probably most importantly, just employing good hygiene and sanitation in the kitchen and properly cooking poultry would destroy any avian influenza virus or other pathogens that might be there.

So while we always need to employ good hygienic practices in the kitchen, we always need to be prepared for an incursion. In fact, the risk this year is no greater, no different than it is and has been every year.

Mr. PETERSON. Thank you.

Thank you, Mr. Chairman.

[The prepared statement of Mr. Peterson follows:]

PREPARED STATEMENT OF HON. COLLIN C. PETERSON, A REPRESENTATIVE IN CONGRESS FROM THE STATE OF MINNESOTA

I would like to thank the chairman for holding this timely hearing and to thank our distinguished witness for joining us today. Minnesota is the largest turkey-growing State in the United States. The value of this important industry exceeds $600 million in Minnesota. So, the concerns being raised about avian influenza could have a major economic impact on my district and on the larger poultry industry.

The Minnesota Turkey Growers Association, in cooperation with veterinarians, APHIS, State, and university officials, has a longstanding and effective avian influenza prevention and control program. I'm confident that the industry and growers are doing everything possible to prepare for the potential for bird flu in Minnesota. However, I am concerned that the introduction of a more virulent strain and factors outside the growers' control may be overwhelming.

I look forward to the comments and information today from Dr. DeHaven on what the USDA is doing to prepare, monitor and possibly execute a program should this dangerous strain, H5N1, find its way into the United States.

The CHAIRMAN. I thank the gentleman.

Dr. DeHaven, I want to make sure that the takeaway message from this hearing today is very clear, and that is the news from poultry about health and food safety is very good news; the consumer does not need to be in any way concerned about the safety of a poultry that they might consume in restaurants, that they might bring home from the supermarket, and as long as they follow the normal safety precautions that are followed to cook food and so on, there is no more danger from poultry today as there is at any other time because this H5N1 virus is not in the United States.

And also, to make it very clear, so far the good news about what is going on even in Asia is that this virus, which is a very, very deadly virus, has not developed in such a way that—it has not mutated to a form that easily transfers from human to human. So as long as your organization is taking the measures to make sure that poultry from these countries where this is a problem is not getting into the United States—and I know that you are—the American public needs to know that poultry that they purchase here in this country is not in any way tainted by that virus. And if that virus does develop into such a fashion that it can mutate into a form that does transfer easily from human to human, we will have, obviously, a very serious problem to address, the United States and elsewhere in the world, but we will also have still the situation where this will be a problem with people associating with other people and not a situation with the consumption of poultry unless American poultry becomes infected by it, in which case your organization, as I understand it—and I will ask you to clarify that—will take very strong measures to eradicate it. And I wonder if you might take a moment to talk about the risks posed by avian influenza as it relates to poultry consumption.

Dr. DeHaven. Well, Mr. Chairman, I would just confirm everything that you said in terms of its accuracy. We have no evidence at this point to support that that Southeast Asian virus, the H5N1 virus, has entered the United States either in birds or in people.

You are also correct in that while there is a concern that that particular virus could mutate and become one that would transmit easily from person to person, that has not yet happened. It is because of that concern that our colleagues on the public health side as well as in the animal health arena, we are diligently preparing should that happen, and appropriately so.

As you alluded to, we do have very good safeguards in place. Back in 2003, when this virus was first identified, we imposed restrictions on the movement of poultry, poultry products and other birds from any of the countries that have been affected by that. We have alerted our Customs and Border Protection colleagues in the Department of Homeland Security to be extra vigilant to look for poultry products or even smuggled products coming from affected countries.

We only allow birds to come into the United States from countries that are not known to be affected, and even those birds must go through a 30-day quarantine period, and while in quarantine they are tested for a number of avian diseases to include avian influenza.

If we were to have an incursion of a low path influenza virus, a highly pathogenic avian influenza, or even this particular H5N1 highly pathogenic virus, we are prepared with an extensive response mechanism. We have been responding to avian influenza for decades in this country; we are just more vigilant than ever with this increased threat represented by this particular virus. So indeed we are prepared to respond on the animal side.

Also, again, I think emphasis on just good food safety in the kitchen, good hygiene practices to eliminate the potential risk that any of the pathoges, whether they be bacterial or virus, might pose, but here again, those ought to be practices that are employed all of the time, every year, and there is no increased risk this year as opposed to any other year.

The CHAIRMAN. Thank you. So we have established that the poultry supply in the United States is today as safe as it has always been. And our next question is then is, what happens if we have a concern that this H5N1, high pathogenic avian influenza, should enter this country? Depopulation will be a necessary step if we do have an outbreak here. When foot-and-mouth disease occurred in Britain, the USDA gave assurances that all necessary funds will be available to quickly depopulate infected herds if the disease entered the United States. Are you able to make a similar statement regarding highly pathogenic avian influenza?

Dr. DeHAVEN. You are correct that if this virus were to enter into the United States, or if we were to get an incursion of any other highly pathogenic virus, the key is early detection and rapid response, and we have those mechanisms in place. As the highly pathogenic avian influenza situation in Texas in 2004 pointed out, we quickly identified that virus and were able to very quickly quarantine the premise, depopulate the birds, do surveillance testing, and assure our trading partners that we had eliminated the virus.

In that situation, as would happen with any incursion of a highly pathogenic virus, we would take those same steps. We would impose quarantines, movement controls, quickly work to eradicate and do surveillance testing in the area. And we would seek emergency funding through the Commodity Credit Corporation source of funds to provide for that kind of response mechanism. Historically we have provided for indemnity and paid for the cleaning and disinfection costs, and with a highly pathogenic virus historically we have paid indemnity at 100 percent of fair market value.

The CHAIRMAN. Thank you.

The gentleman from Colorado Mr. Salazar is recognized.

Mr. SALAZAR. Thank you, Mr. Chairman.

I understand that on November 1, 2005, the President actually submitted a request to Congress for the $7.1 billion in emergency funding, and of that, $91 million I guess is going to USDA. Could you expound as to how that money is going to be utilized, please?

Dr. DeHAVEN. Indeed. Of the $91 million, $91.35 million to be exact, that was targeted for the USDA, about $18.3 million would go towards efforts internationally, and the balance, $73 million would go towards domestic activities.

For our international activities, much of it would involve surveillance in poultry, commercial poultry, wildlife and even swine, some $8 million going towards that effort.

I will just hit on the high points of some of the activities that we had in mind. $2.1 million would go to in-country expertise where we would provide expertise both in laboratory diagnosis, operations related to vaccination and eradication of the virus, as well as just overall response mechanisms. We would suggest putting teams of experts, consultants, in those countries, if you will, to provide them in-country expertise to help with their response mechanism, recognizing again that by reducing the virus load in the affected countries, we, if not eliminate, certainly reduce the potential and delay the potential for this particular virus to mutate to one that could easily spread from people to people.

A million dollars would go towards training and education in proper destruction and response mechanisms to an outbreak.

Of the $73 million that is identified for domestic purposes, $10 million would be used for cooperative agreements, for sample collection and additional surveillance; $3 million for additional people to do some of that domestic surveillance activities, both in our live bird markets as well as in our commercial industry; $3 million for additional diagnostic capability at our laboratories, and for the reagents that would need to be on hand to do the additional level of testing; $17 million for wild bird surveillance in the Alaska and other North American flyways, and that would be done in concert with our colleagues in the Department of Interior; $10 million for stockpiling of vaccine and supplies and materials that might be needed for a response to this H5N1 virus in the United States; $7 million to organize, train and equip State management response teams as well as our reserve corps. We have a corps of some 700 veterinarians and 500 animal health technicians who have identified their willingness to volunteer to assist us if we were to have that outbreak situation; $7 million to our agricultural research service, working with their partners both at the Federal and State level for research in methods development, improved vaccine and biosecurity measures; and $9 million directed towards smuggling interdiction, to try and find products that people may be attempting to enter the United States with products that would potentially carry a risk of bringing the virus here.

Mr. SALAZAR. Thank you, Mr. Chairman. I yield back.

The CHAIRMAN. The gentleman from Kansas Mr. Moran is recognized.

Mr. MORAN. Mr. Chairman, thank you very much. Thank you for holding this hearing. Certainly this is a topic of great importance and receiving a lot of attention across the country, including in Kansas.

Concerns about our border are clearly evident. Your testimony indicates that discussions have occurred—the Department of Homeland Security personnel have been instructed what to look for, and I think your word is a valiant effort. Tell me about how our border is closed to potential infected animals, birds, and how successful confident you are in your statement about the valiant efforts.

Dr. DeHAVEN. Well, some of the safeguards we have in place, Congressman Moran, include the fact that back in 2003, when this virus was first identified in Southeast Asia, we immediately imposed import restrictions on poultry, poultry products and birds from affected countries. So that has been in place for nearly 2 years now.

To implement that, we alert, of course, Customs and Border Protections within DHS to those concerns, and as it relates to poultry or poultry products that might be coming to our borders, they are actually the enforcement agency.

Within APHIS, we have some 50 veterinarians at our ports and borders, veterinarians that are with our Veterinary Services Unit, in addition to 13 veterinarians with our Plant Protection and Quarantine Unit who work side by side with our border protection colleagues to ensure that those restrictions are actually being imposed at our ports and borders. There have been a number of written alerts as we find additional countries affected, emphasizing the need to continue those restrictions as well as add additional countries for those restrictions.

Mr. MORAN. Have restricted birds been found at the border and detained, killed, destroyed?

Dr. DEHAVEN. Indeed. A couple of weeks ago we did find 100 baby chicks from Vietnam at the Dallas-Ft. Worth airport. They were caught by our Customs and Border Protection colleagues and appropriately destroyed.

Mr. MORAN. Doctor, could you describe for me what you think is the most logical or likely scenario of this avian influenza, its development not only in the United States, but around the world; what do you forsee the future to look like?

Dr. DEHAVEN. Well, there is a lot of speculation being done by a lot of experts both on the animal health as well as the public health side about the likelihood or the possibility that this particular virus will mutate and become one that is easily transmitted from human to human. The fact that we have several countries in the world affected by a highly pathogenic virus, one that is highly pathogenic to birds, is enough for us to be very, very concerned, whether it ever does or does not mutate to a pandemic-type virus. So we have appropriate safeguards in place. We have bolstered those safeguards because of this situation, and obviously because of the potential for this virus to mutate.

I would hesitate to speculate on whether or not this virus or another one might mutate and become a pandemic. I think it is only prudent that we prepare for that, we prepare for the worst, hope for the best, and I think that is the strategy that we are employing, and is the strategy that is laid out in the President's National Strategy that he laid out on November 1st.

Mr. MORAN. Doctor, is there a time frame in which one would know whether the virus would mutate? If this doesn't happen by a certain point in time, it is not going to happen, or this is a fear that we would have now into the future?

Dr. DEHAVEN. As long as the virus is out there and circulating, it has the potential to mutate. And it is like a roll of the dice, if you will, as to whether it happens 2 days from now, 2 months from now, 2 years from now or forever. But as long as the virus is circulating, circulating in birds, it has the potential to mutate. That is why it is important, as we prepare for a pandemic, that we also work with those veterinary officials in those countries affected to contain and reduce, if not eliminate, that virus. The only way we will eliminate the potential for this to become a pandemic is to eliminate the virus in birds, and that is why we are focusing efforts on working with those countries to attack the virus at its source.

Mr. MORAN. Are all the countries cooperating with us in this effort? Are there those that are less cooperative than they should be or need to be?

Dr. DEHAVEN. I think because of the potential magnitude of this problem, the overall cooperation internationally is very good, and that was clearly evident at the meeting I attended sponsored by a number of international organizations. So the cooperation with those international organizations has been good. I think the transparency has been quite good relative to what we might otherwise expect in terms of countries reporting incidents of the virus in their poultry. So I think it has been better than what typically we would expect in terms of willingness and desire to cooperate, as well as transparency.

Mr. MORAN. Dr. DeHaven, thank you very much for answering my questions, but also thank you for efforts in this regard. You have a reputation of someone that I am pleased to see in the position that you are in at the time that we face. Thank you.

Dr. DEHAVEN. Thank you very much.

The CHAIRMAN. I thank the gentleman.

The gentleman from North Dakota, Mr. Pomeroy, is recognized.

Mr. POMEROY. I thank the Chair. I want to thank the Chair especially for holding this hearing, and the construction of the chairman's comments.

I think it is important that we try to understand all of this in perspective. I remember getting my swine flu shot until that program was stopped. We understood the shots were killing more than the flu.

And as we evaluate this one, the President has now committed a multibillion-dollar response, and I am glad he did. But can you just give us kind of the general view in terms of what has led us to make this kind of commitment; how do we see this threat warranting this type of response at this time? And yet—I guess you have emphasized throughout your testimony this morning the absence of this virus with U.S. poultry means that at present we are very well positioned, especially heading into the holiday season, in terms of any concerns the public might have about the consumption of poultry. And then I have a follow-up question.

Dr. DEHAVEN. Certainly, thank you.

First of all, the fact that we have a virus that is circulating in a number of countries in Southeast Asia and now Eastern Europe, a virus that is highly pathogenic to poultry, is enough of a reason for my agency to increase its safeguards, bolster the measures that we already have in place to safeguard the United States, as well as ensure that we have appropriate response mechanisms in place to respond if that poultry virus should enter the United States.

Mr. POMEROY. Is there an evaluation in terms of how it is spreading in those affected areas?

Dr. DEHAVEN. There has been a lot of speculation about how it has been spreading. Some of the spread is consistent with what is known about the migratory bird pass; that, in fact, some of it could be being spread by migratory birds. It is also just as likely that some of the spread is occurring because of people, equipment, poultry or poultry products, or other birds that may be moving perhaps illegally. So it is hard to definitively determine, but clearly migratory birds as well as the ongoing day-to-day international movement of people and products is potential.

Mr. POMEROY. Are there things about poultry production there that are different than here that are making the spread more likely?

Dr. DEHAVEN. I think that the poultry production in those countries varies widely from commercial production that is consistent and comparable to the level of production and the type of production that we see in our commercial industry to some countries where the only industry is the individual producer who has his own flock or menagerie of birds that he is raising for his own purposes and perhaps selling some of those birds at a local market. So I think what we are seeing runs the gamut. As we have in this country, our ability to respond is largely the ability of our commercial industry to work us with, good biosecurity to limit the spread, ability to provide an appropriate response mechanism, whether that be vaccination or depopulation, et cetera.

When you have a number of individuals operating independently, when you are identifying infected flocks and perhaps destroying those birds without providing that producer any compensation, it makes it difficult to find all of the potential infection and——

Mr. POMEROY. Is some of the USDA activity in providing aid and assistance to other countries in terms of how they might develop perhaps more effective strategies that—poultry production basically, and then certainly disease containment?

Dr. DEHAVEN. Indeed, Congressman Pomeroy, that has been our efforts thus far, and that is what we want to expand upon or would expand upon if the money that the President has requested is approved, working with those countries in terms of assessing what their needs are and what is the best strategy. In some countries the best strategy may be depopulation. In other countries it may be so widespread or the infrastructure so lacking that vaccination would be the best strategy, and in some countries a combination of depopulation and vaccination might be appropriate.

Mr. POMEROY. I found the book, "The Great Influenza, The Epic Story of the Deadliest Fight in History", by John Barry, to be very interesting and a wonderful description of how the flu virus mutates. And it is almost a given, from my understanding of the book, and I am certainly not a scientist, that the prevalence of this virus is going to make mutation inevitable, and mutation may or may not make this significantly more contagious. But as I understand the present state of this thing, it is highly contagious within poultry, not terribly contagious from poultry to human, and not—if humans, because of their extraordinarily close contact with poultry, get this virus, they have not been highly contagious to other humans; is that about the state of play right now?

Dr. DEHAVEN. My understanding is the same as yours. Certainly I can confirm the ability of this virus to spread very rapidly from bird to bird, and it would appear that those humans who have become infected with this virus have had close contact with infected birds, and little or no spread from person to person.

What makes this virus unique, however, is the fact that it does affect humans. I mentioned that since 1924 we have had three incursions of highly pathogenic AI into the United States. None of those three involved a virus that produced significant disease in humans. The human health issue was not really a concern. So what makes this particular virus unique is that it not only causes high mortality in birds, it has the potential to kill people, and we have seen that.

So if this particular virus that can kill people also mutates and gains the ability to spread rapidly from person to person, then we have the real concern.

By reducing the virus load, by reducing the virus interactions or the potential for the virus to interact and mutate, we reduce the potential for it to mutate into this pathogenic virus. The best way to do that is to reduce the virus load in the affected poultry in those countries. That is why we need to, as we prepare for a pandemic, also attack the virus at its source and thereby eliminate or reduce the potential for the virus to become a pandemic-type virus.

Mr. POMEROY. Thank you for your helpful testimony.

Thank you, Mr. Chairman.

The CHAIRMAN. I thank the gentleman.

It is my pleasure to recognize the gentleman from North Carolina, the chairman of the Livestock Subcommittee who has been very interested in this matter and has a good deal of poultry in his congressional district as well, Mr. Hayes.

Mr. HAYES. Thank you, Mr. Chairman, I appreciate you holding the hearing today. And I point out a couple of things. As you have alluded to, I think Virginia is No. 10, North Carolina is No. 3 in poultry, so a vitally important issue. And I would ask unanimous consent to submit my opening statement for the record.

The CHAIRMAN. Without objection.

[The prepared statement of Mr. Hayes follows:]

PREPARED STATEMENT OF HON. ROBIN HAYES, A REPRESENTATIVE IN CONGRESS FROM THE STATE OF NORTH CAROLINA

I want to thank Chairman Goodlatte for holding this timely hearing so that the committee may review the U.S. Department of Agriculture's responsibilities related to the prevention, detection, and eradication of avian influenza (AI). North Carolina is the Nation's third largest poultry-producing state and the threat of Asian-type avian influenza in poultry should be taken seriously. I am hopeful this hearing will bring to light some key facts about the disease and USDA's efforts to prevent its introduction to the United States.

The type of AI now occurring in Southeast Asia is called H5NI, a highly pathogenic avian influenza strain. USDA has stated that the United States. has never had an outbreak of Asian-type H5N1, and we do not have any cases now.

I know the U.S. has multiple lines of defense against Asian H5N1. The importation of birds or bird products from the affected area overseas has been harmed or placed under strict control by the U.S. Government. Experience in the past indicates migratory patterns of birds that affect Asia do not generally make their way to the U.S., although scientists check migratory birds to look for signs that wild birds might carry the virus to the United States. Surveillance testing in commercial poultry flocks is also ongoing. USDA is working with international experts and organizations to assist affected countries and neighboring countries with disease prevention, management, and eradication activities. By helping these countries, USDA can reduce the risk of the disease spreading from overseas to the United States. Additionally, President Bush took a proactive stance by unveiling the National Strategy to Safeguard Against the Danger of Pandemic Influenza.

AI is a threat that needs full attention by Federal and State regulatory agencies and the poultry industry, but fear should not turn into mass hysteria. With vigilant safeguards in place, surveillance testing underway and proper biosecurity measures, I believe that from an agricultural perspective we are on the right path to prepare for this disease.

Mr. Chairman, I appreciate you holding this hearing so we can learn more about USDA's efforts to prevent Asian-type H5NI from reaching the United States and how USDA is monitoring for the disease. Should it reach our shores, USDA needs to be fully prepared to contain and eradicate the disease. I look forward to Dr. DeHaven's testimony today.

Mr. HAYES. Mr. DeHaven, North Carolina has been very active, particularly in the area of poultry in the mail. We had some issues here potentially with the avian influenza that are quite disturbing, and I appreciate your effort to work with us to cover that base.

Can you elaborate on that just a moment for us while we look at these different issues?

Dr. DeHAVEN. Certainly. Part of our efforts are to look at all potential pathways of not only virus introduction, but, once it is introduced, ways that it might spread. And as you are alluding to, there are a large number of birds, primarily commercial chicks, young chicks that are moved by the U.S. Postal Service every day. There is no mandatory testing requirement for any birds that might be moved that way; however, as I indicated, most of them are coming from commercial operations where there is some level of surveillance.

Having said that, we are looking at that as a potential pathway, and also looking at ways that we might mitigate whatever risk that it would represent. This is a practice that has been going on for a number of years. It only involves domestic poultry. We are not talking about the Postal Service bringing in birds from other countries, but rather the movement of birds within the United States. Nevertheless, were we to have a virus, high-path virus, or any other, for that matter, in the United States, this is a potential pathway for spread, and so one that we are carefully evaluating now and looking at ways we might mitigate that risk without unduly restricting movement of birds.

Mr. HAYES. I look forward to working with you on that as the poultry folks are interested, obviously as well, working on some way to have the proper paperwork to prevent that happening.

Two questions together. In the agriculture appropriations bill in 2005, $23 million was provided for the influenza program. Talk a little bit about how this money is being spent. Particularly given the idea that there is some misinformation out there, we want to reassure the public as to the safety of consumption of properly prepared cooked poultry. And then in cooperation with the States, describe how we are working to educate producers in the issues that we are talking about here today.

Dr. DeHAVEN. With regard to the $23 million appropriation for low-pathogenic avian influenza, approximately half of that money was set aside for indemnity. Should we have an incursion of an H5 or an H7 low-path avian influenza virus, those monies would be used to indemnify producers whose flocks would be affected by that.

The balance of that is to increase our overall surveillance program in the United States, both in our live bird markets, best known to the northeast part of the country, as well as increased surveillance in our commercial operations.

As for the commercial side, we are working through the long-standing National Poultry Improvement Plan or NPIP, an organization that includes industry representation. And the efforts there are to increase the already significant surveillance that is in place for avian influenza, and I might stress avian influenza of all types, particularly low-path H5, H7, obviously any testing would also find a highly pathogenic virus.

We are also concentrating a lot of effort in the live bird markets, initially in the northeast, but we are working to extend that to a number of States such as California that also have live bird markets.

In the Northeast we have on a regular basis found an H5 or H7 virus in those markets. We now have in place uniform procedures where—in New York and New Jersey in particular, where the majority of those live bird markets are in the Northeast, birds have to be tested before they get there. We are testing at least on a quarterly basis those live bird markets, and should we find the virus, they are shut down, cleaned, and disinfected, and any birds that would be present properly disposed of. And this is what we are working on expanding to other parts of the country.

So we in essence are creating a low-path H5 H7 avian influenza program, and that is largely in response to, one, recognition that those two subtypes have shown the ability in the past to mutate to high path; and second, to be consistent with the international standard just put in place by the OIE, that recognizes low-path H5 and H7 as notifiable diseases.

Mr. HAYES. Thank you, sir.

Mr. Chairman, I have one more question, but I will yield back and wait for the next round.

The CHAIRMAN. Go ahead.

Mr. HAYES. Under the new OIE guidelines you explain that trade restrictions should be limited to the affected zone or region rather than banning products from an entire country. You mentioned that USDA would do this in response to regionalization requests from another country. I was wondering if any of the affected countries in Southeast Asia have asked to be regionalized and what is USDA's response?

Dr. DEHAVEN. You are correct in that the OIE does recognize the concept of regionalization where a country can be affected, but portions of that country can be certified by a potential importing country as free of the disease. In fact, the OIE has taken that concept of regionalization one step further, calling it compartmentalization, recognizing that there may be a compartment. It may be—for example, a compartment could be a live bird market or the live bird market system. A compartment could be one integrated poultry company and the virus hasn't affected others.

So we would, and have in the past, whenever we have an incursion of avian influenza, worked with our trading partners to regionalize the U.S., only impose restrictions on the affected parts of the country and let trade continue unrestricted from the other parts of the country. And we will employ this compartmentalization as well in the future should it apply.

Because of the widespread nature of the virus in Southeast Asia and in many of those countries, the lack of the infrastructure to effectively deal with it, no country has yet requested that we regionalize them for this disease. Certainly if we were to receive such a request we would respond accordingly. But just from the 50,000-

foot level, and speaking regionally rather than by a country-by-country level, the virus does not seem to be well contained enough yet where we could recognize a portion of a country free. Again, should we receive such a request, we would carefully consider it.

Mr. HAYES. Thank you very much. And if we do, and we consider it, make sure it is a reciprocal agreement.

Thank you, Mr. Chairman.

The CHAIRMAN. I thank the gentleman.

The gentleman from Pennsylvania, Mr. Holden, is recognized.

Mr. HOLDEN. Thank you, Mr. Chairman.

Doctor, thank you for your testimony and your very knowledgeable answers to the questions that have been put forth to you.

I would just like to follow up on Mr. Salazar's question about the funding. I believe you stated that USDA will receive about $90 million out of the $7.1 million that has been proposed by the President to address the problem, and you highlighted and explained in detail what you plan to do with that, and I commend you for that. And maybe you are not the appropriate person to ask this question, but where is the other $7 billion that the President asked for going to be directed to combat this problem?

Dr. DEHAVEN. Most of those monies—and I will let it in a very general statement—most of those monies would go towards the public health agencies to prepare for a pandemic, a human avian influenza pandemic virus; such things as developing and stockpiling an effective vaccine, stockpiling antiviral medications, that sort of thing.

I think it is prudent, though, that I point out while $91 million would go to the Department of Agriculture for our efforts, we are only one country out of a broad international community that is willing and anxious to attack this virus at its source, in the birds. Our efforts would be directed through those international organizations to help. So while our $91 million is a significant sum, there are other funding sources, other countries, who are willing and anxious to participate in that effort as well.

So again, it is a two-pronged strategy where we work to prepare for a pandemic while we also work to attack the virus at its source and reduce the likelihood that we will have a pandemic.

Mr. HOLDEN. And the $91 million you feel is sufficient for the concerns you have to address?

Dr. DEHAVEN. Again, because the United States is only one source of potential funding, it will help us bolster our domestic efforts while we also work internationally, in concert with other international sources of funding. It will go a long way towards assisting in that overall effort.

Mr. HOLDEN. One question, Doctor. I have several chicken farms and at least one large duck farm in my district in Pennsylvania. And since ducks do not usually show symptoms of avian influenza, if they do carry it, can you tell us more about monitoring for the virus in ducks and other domestic water fowl?

Dr. DEHAVEN. In fact, Pennsylvania in particular has a good surveillance program in place. Some of those ducks for that matter are going to the live bird markets in New Jersey and New York where there is a requirement that they be tested.

So we don't have a surveillance program specific to ducks but, rather, any animals that would be moving interstate would be subject to some level of testing.

With the additional monies that the President is requesting in this program, we would expand our domestic surveillance, not just with commercial chickens and poultry, but with other species of birds as well.

I would point out that while there clearly are some ducks that have shown to be asymptomatic carriers—they can have the virus without being affected by it—that is not always the case, and clearly that is not the case with all migratory birds. So while we would emphasize as well in terms of seeing if the virus is getting close by testing migratory birds, any evidence of migratory bird die-off, ducks or other species, would be a good indication that we need to take a closer look and do some additional testing.

Mr. HOLDEN. Thank you, Doctor. I yield back.

The CHAIRMAN. I thank the gentleman.

The gentlewoman from Colorado, Ms. Musgrave, is recognized.

Mrs. MUSGRAVE. Thank you, Mr. Chairman.

Dr. DeHaven, can you speak to us about surveillance of migratory birds? I am looking at these flyways, and it looks like a very daunting task to try to do that. Could you tell us how it is done, please?

Dr. DeHAVEN. I will, indeed. There has been some level of migratory bird surveillance in the United States ongoing since 1998 in the Alaska flyway. And indeed, the most likely route of bringing the virus to the United States from migratory birds would be through that Alaska or Pacific flyway. The reason for that is that there are other populations of birds in Asia that part of their migratory path takes them over Siberia and Alaska, as do our migratory birds. So in theory, you could have a migratory bird from Asia that is infected, could encounter, interact with, and subsequently infect a migratory bird from North America in that Alaska flyway, and that bird could bring it, in theory, to the United States. Probably a remote possibility, but nevertheless it could happen.

Not knowing exactly how birds might or might not migrate, as well as just to be vigilant, there are a number of migratory bird pathways, as you indicate, in North America. Part of the money that the President has requested, $17 million would go towards doing wild bird surveillance on all of those migratory bird pathways. We think that while that is just one potential pathway for bringing the virus to the United States—and some would argue not a very likely pathway—regardless, in the context of being thorough and vigilant, we would with those monies do increased surveillance in all of those pathways with our colleagues in Department of Interior, who have really the legislative authority to do that kind of a program, as well as the expertise.

Mrs. MUSGRAVE. So you would work with the Department of Interior.

Dr. DeHAVEN. Indeed. We already have been working with them in terms of designing a potential migratory bird pathway or Migratory Bird Pathway Surveillance Program, one that would actually commence this spring.

Mrs. MUSGRAVE. OK. Thank you very much.

The CHAIRMAN. I thank the gentlewoman. The gentlewoman from South Dakota, Ms. Herseth, is recognized.

Ms. HERSETH. Thank you, Mr. Chairman. Thank you to you, Mr. Peterson, for this very important hearing.

And Dr. DeHaven, I too would like to commend you for your testimony today and your helpful responses to the questions of my colleagues.

I would also like to follow up on some of the funding issues here and how the portion of the President's request that would go to the USDA would be used.

You mentioned in your testimony that USDA would like to stockpile additional animal vaccine. Can you talk at a little bit more length about the state of our current supply of the vaccine and where you feel that the additional stockpiles would be helpful in inoculation of birds in this country, and just how much we are looking at in the production capacity for the vaccine?

Dr. DEHAVEN. We do, in fact, already have a potential vaccine bank for avian influenza. Again, because of the potential for the H5 and H7 subtypes to mutate to highly pathogenic avian influenza, the bank we currently have includes 40 million doses of vaccine, 20 million each for H5 and H7. And this was a stockpile that we had in place long before, or had contemplated long before the current situation with the H5N1 virus in Southeast Asia.

I would point out, however, that our colleagues in the Agricultural Research Service have done challenge studies with this vaccine against the virus in Asia and it does provide very good protection to birds against that particular virus. Now, again, that would just be half of the bank that we have, and the other half is H7. So, the 20 million doses of H5 vaccine we have in place would be effective.

We also, with the 2006 appropriation now in place, will proceed with purchasing an additional 30 million doses of H5 and H7. So that would give us 70 million. With the emergency funding request by the President, 10 million would go towards additional vaccine. That would buy us an additional 40 million doses of strictly H5 vaccine that we could use for this particular virus.

So we have a supply on hand readily. Vaccination would not ordinarily be one of the tools that we would first use if we were to have an incursion, but to the extent that we had a widespread incursion or again just based on the circumstances we may use it to ring vaccinate around infection, for example. It is in the toolbox if we need it, and the additional funding would provide us the ability to substantially literally double the number we currently have on hand.

Avian influenza viruses are something that are used commercially internationally, so the capacity to produce vaccine internationally for birds is there, and we don't feel that there would be a shortage in the short-term to produce additional vaccine should it be needed.

Ms. HERSETH. Thank you for the comprehensiveness of your answer to some of my follow-up questions there.

Let me ask one other question. In South Dakota, we have a growing turkey industry, as well as one of the largest goose farms in the country. And I know in response to some other questions you indicated that we are looking at a lot of different species here in the approach of the USDA to prepare and protect different producers from the threat of avian flu.

Now, you had also mentioned, I think in response to Mr. Peterson's question, that last year USDA spent approximately $4 million in a biosecurity campaign. In any of the 2006 appropriations or in the President's request would you have some follow-up to that in terms of outreach to producers around the country as a follow-up to that campaign for this year?

I am a little concerned if that was money expended last year, what the follow-up has been in outreach this year, particularly with the public attention and the threat and the risk that is perceived to be out there. And maybe that is part of what you described as the cooperative agreements or increase in domestic surveillance.

Dr. DEHAVEN. That campaign we had a year or two ago called Biosecurity for the Birds was somewhere in excess of $4 million and resulted in the production of a number of outreach materials, brochures, compact disks, public announcements, and in multiple languages as well. Much of the cost associated with that kind of outreach campaign is developing those materials. So the materials that we have are as relevant today for the current threat as they were when they were produced. So we would benefit from already having those materials available that we could simply increase production and distribution of and, indeed, have those materials in a number of languages and have talked already about putting them in some of the languages found in Southeast Asia to help those countries.

In the President's request for emergency funding is $1 million for education and outreach, particularly in live bird markets. But here again, whether we are reaching out to live bird markets to other countries or to commercial production, many of those materials that are outreach efforts would be equally useful in a number of different venues.

Ms. HERSETH. Thank you very much, Doctor. I yield back.

The CHAIRMAN. I thank the gentlewoman.

The gentleman from Minnesota, Mr. Gutknecht, is recognized.

Mr. GUTKNECHT. Thank you, Mr. Chairman.

Thank you, Dr. DeHaven. You have been an articulate voice for sound science and common sense for a long time, and as one member I would like to publicly thank you for that.

I want to talk a little bit about sound science and common sense. Now, this is not the Budget Committee, and I served on the Budget Committee for 8 years. I want to take a second here for the benefit of Members to note that on October 31 the Food and Agriculture Organization of the World Health Organization proposed $140 million for international response to the current avian influenza outbreak. The very next day the President called for $7.1 billion.

Now, I just think the Congress and the American people are willing to spend whatever it takes, but I just want to say as one member that I think we have to defend on common sense and sound science what it is we are going to try to do. The reason I say that, Dr. DeHaven, is I am afraid what we may end up doing is replicating an awful lot of research already being done in the United

States, and let me give you two examples which you may be aware of.

I will give you a couple of examples. I was in Lubbock, TX, a few weeks ago and visited the ag school at Texas Tech, and there is a professor there, and I do not know if he is correct or not, but he said that he believes there may be a correlation between these kinds of flu viruses and a lack of selenium in the diet of poultry. It seems to me that for a relatively small investment we could find out whether or not that is correct.

Let me give you a couple of other examples. There is a little lab, well, it is not so little, they have some of the most advanced technology that I have ever seen in Worthington, MN, called Newport Labs. This is a group of veterinarians that consult with large producers of livestock around North America. Essentially, what they do is if an animal, whether it be a bird or a pig or beef cattle, or whatever it happens to be, if one of them gets sick, they use a cotton swab, they put it in a test tube, they FedEx it overnight to Worthington, MN, and they have the technology in this lab to do, I think the term is CPR or CRP, whatever it is, they replicate the genetic makeup very, very quickly. Bottom line is that within 24 hours they will have the correct vaccine on its way back to that rancher or producer.

This is happening today in real time, and it is happening in the private sector. And the other example I wanted to share with you is something I was made aware of about 8 months ago. I got a tour of some of the labs that a little medical practice started by the Mayo brothers in my hometown of Rochester, MN, and they are already—in fact this was 8 months ago—they had already, using the information that was available to them, using their supercomputer, had essentially showed us a three-dimensional representation of what they thought this particular flu virus would look like.

Now, that was interesting, but what was even more interesting, using this supercomputer they had literally taken what they thought would be the 10 most likely vaccines to use against this virus, and at least on a computer model had determined which one they thought would be most effective.

The reason I mention all this is because I think you are in a unique position to be helpful, and because I just hope we don't throw money at the problem like that one commercial we see right now, where King Arthur says, "You mean we should throw money at the problem?" and the consultant says, "Precisely." I hope we don't wind up ignoring some of the really good research going on at universities and at labs. Not only at places like Mayo Clinic, but more importantly like little labs in Worthington, Minnesota, called Newport Labs.

So we have worked together on some of the other issues before. In fact, I think we have reported to you some interesting things being done at another little lab, and you have been working with them. So if you want to respond to that, you can, but I just wanted to make certain we make that part of the public record.

Dr. DeHaven. Thank you, Congressman, and I am indeed aware of the study that was done with regard to selenium and the ability of selenium and diet to provide some resistance to virus.

As you might guess, for example, during the BSE situation, we had a number of individuals and companies and academics, private sector as well as university settings, that had the cure-all for BSE. We need to take those comments seriously, give them all due consideration, and indeed the ability of selenium to provide some degree of immunity or resistance is one of those areas we need to carefully look at.

We have, in fact, taken advantage of some of the previous situations, the low-path avian influenza situation in Virginia, for example, to develop a PCR test, a rapid test for detecting avian influenza. We now have 36 State laboratories that are trained and certified to run that test should we need to be able to do so.

So we have in fact taken advantage of technology produced in the private sector or produced elsewhere and employed those technologies in our programs. Our colleagues in CSREES and ARS obviously are involved in research, and they have a good research network with academic institutions. And indeed, it was ARS's Southeast Poultry Research Laboratory, working with concert with the University of Alaska, that has been doing the migratory bird surveillance.

So those partnerships exist, and I couldn't agree with you more that, one, we need to take advantage of them and make every good use of the technology that is out there, recognizing that some of these great ideas are nothing more than a great idea and others potentially have tremendous application.

The CHAIRMAN. I thank the gentleman.

The gentleman from Washington, Mr. Larsen, is recognized.

Mr. LARSEN. Thank you, Mr. Chairman.

Dr. DeHaven, a couple of questions. First, on the issue of testing.

Basically, the first question I have is, are there resources available for testing labs, such as those located in my State, Washington State University, to get access to what is called high-throughput testing?

Dr. DEHAVEN. This would be the PCR testing that I mentioned, where we develop the test as a result of or during the low-path AI situation in Virginia a couple of years ago.

We have 36 State laboratories that have been trained, certified, and will be proficiency tested in doing that testing. I can't tell you off the top of my head if we have the laboratory in Washington State approved or not. Certainly, Terry McElwain, the director of that laboratory, and his reputation and the reputation of that laboratory are well-known within those circles, and Terry does a lot of testing for us.

I suspect if he had an interest in, if not already approved, and I do not know that it is not, I am sure we could arrange that.

Mr. LARSEN. Thanks. In the spring of 2004, following the outbreak of the avian flu in British Columbia, APHIS sent a number of personnel to Wahkiakum County to monitor the outbreak. Wahkiakum is in my district and it is on the border with British Columbia, shares the border, and I want to thank APHIS for their quick work in responding to that outbreak and APHIS has been helpful in assisting the State Department of Agriculture to develop plans to step up surveillance and safety measures to protect against potential infection.

One of the things I discussed with your folks when I visited was the fact that at the time I think they were set up to be sort of an emergency deployment crew, if you will. I think the gentleman who is heading the effort in Wahkiakum County was from Kansas, if I am not mistaken. The question I had of him, and he did not have the answer, is whether or not we were trying to make that kind of deployment crew permanent, like a permanent SWAT team, as opposed to we need one so you come from here, and you come from here, and you come from here, and we are going to send you all to this place.

Have you or is there an idea that you may want to try to make that more of a permanent capacity within APHIS?

Dr. DeHAVEN. Historically, our animal disease emergency response capability has been regionally based, and when we had four regions we had four SWAT teams, as you say, or four response teams. A number of years ago, when we moved into two regions, we only had two.

We started to do some computer modeling looking at the potential threats from a number of areas and a number of different diseases and realized a regional response just would not be adequate if we were to deal with an introduction of a highly contagious disease that in fact may be present in 5 or 10 or 35 States at any given time. So we have been working over the past decade diligently to move our level of response from a regional response to a State level response so that we would have typically the State veterinarian and our area veterinarian in charge, our senior Federal veterinarian, would be codirectors for a State response mechanism.

Indeed, those response teams now exist in every State of the Union. They work on the incident command structure that every emergency response organization, whether they be forest firefighters or emergency disaster response mechanisms, would use. So we have the same jargon, the same structure, but the difference is we now have that capability at the State level.

We have mandatory training that every employee in APHIS be trained in incident command response, because virtually every employee in our agency is a first responder. The concept is the State veterinarian and the AVIC in the affected States would codirect a State response coordinated regionally and then nationally. When we have personnel in a part of the country that is not affected, they become resources for those teams in States that are affected.

So what you saw in Washington, as we prepared for and responded to that avian influenza situation in British Columbia, we could basically provide in every State.

Mr. LARSEN. And because of this border issue, how do you coordinate with BC and Canadian authorities in that case?

Dr. DeHAVEN. In fact, we have close coordination with them, in that we have a North American Animal Health Committee that is made up of animal health officials from Canada, Mexico, and the United States. We have recently concluded a series of three or four test exercises where we exercise cross-border disease outbreaks in two countries or in three countries. We have shared each other's response mechanism structures with each other, and they are very similar, and we have written agreements where in fact if one country is affected we will share people and resources across the border to help with an outbreak in another country.

So I think the cross-border cooperation is very, very good. And of course with the BSE situation, we have had lots of opportunity to work across the border with our friends and colleagues in Canada.

Mr. LARSEN. Right. Well, thank you, Dr. DeHaven. I will follow up with your staff on the Washington State University.

Dr. DeHAVEN. Thank you.

Mr. LARSEN. Thank you. Thank you, Mr. Chairman.

The CHAIRMAN. I thank the gentleman.

The gentlewoman from Ohio, Mrs. Schmidt, is recognized.

Mrs. SCHMIDT. Thank you, Mr. Chairman, and thank you, Doctor, for being here.

In my district, while much of it is an agricultural district, poultry is a small portion of it, a very small portion. But the economic impact of that is a $14 million impact a year. About 150 people are directly employed in the poultry side of it, and we don't even have a large poultry plant. So from an economic side, this is a very serious issue across the United States because these are just simple little cottage farmers that have a few chickens that have a $14 million impact. And of course, the risk to the elderly and other fragile portions of the population would create an enormous health risk to the United States.

So having those issues at hand, my question to you is a threefold question: In developing your Avian Influenza Surveillance Plan, how do you conduct sampling to monitor the conditions of the Nation's flock? Is it targeted or random? How do you determine where the samples are taken and how many? And who actually collects the samples, and then what do you do with them afterwards?

Dr. DeHAVEN. We share a very, very good working relationship with the poultry industry across the country. And much of the testing program that we have in place is based upon that cooperative relationship. Having good surveillance in place is mutually beneficial to us.

We have a number of mechanisms for achieving active surveillance as opposed to passive surveillance. Through our National Poultry Improvement Plan we are monitoring virtually every breeding flock in the country. We have an AI, Avian Influenza, Clean Program for those breeding flocks where there is required testing for participation in that program, and those samples are collected by the industry but tested at laboratories that our Federal National Poultry Improvement Program have approved.

We have mandatory testing of flocks for any poultry products that may be eligible for export. Obviously, all of our major poultry companies are producing some product for export, and there is some required testing for any poultry products or from poultry where the meat may be destined for export. Those samples are again collected by the industry but tested at State-approved laboratories.

Any movement of birds to the live bird markets, particularly those in New York and New Jersey, where we have some 80 live bird markets in New York, 35 in New Jersey, they are requiring as a condition of entering those markets that they have a negative test for avian influenza.

States where there have been low-path AI problems in the past, have some State level of testing requirement where those tests are either collected by State personnel or by industry and then tested in State approved laboratories.

Then the industry itself has available to it some rapid test, Directagen being one, where they can do screening tests, and if anything shows up positive, report that to a State laboratory. When it is all said and done, we are testing somewhere in excess of 1.5 million samples a year for avian influenza.

As we develop our Low-Path Avian Influenza Program, and hope soon to publish a proposed rule, with the additional testing that would be part of that program, we would anticipate that level of testing on an annual basis to go up from 1.5 million or more to as much as 4 million samples a year.

I think it is also prudent to point out that if we are talking about the highly pathogenic avian influenza virus, and in particular the Southeast Asia H5N1 virus, it kills birds in large percentages. So our industry is acutely sensitive to any increase in mortality in their commercial flocks. That is something that would be reported very quickly, and that precisely was the case of the high-path outbreak in Texas in 2004.

Mrs. SCHMIDT. Thank you.

The CHAIRMAN. I thank the gentlewoman.

Before I recognize the gentleman from California, Mr. Costa, Dr. DeHaven, let me say I am going to have to leave to go to another meeting, but I want to thank you for your help today in educating the committee on the animal health issues associated with avian influenza. Your insights have been most helpful in framing this issue, and we look forward to working with you as this situation develops.

Finally, with Thanksgiving fast approaching, I would like to take this opportunity to remind everyone that a properly prepared turkey is still the best way to enjoy this traditional holiday meal and will be the highlight of the Goodlatte family gathering in the Sixth Congressional District of Virginia, the largest poultry producing district in the United States.

So I thank you for your help today in educating the public and this committee about what risks are out there and how we are dealing with them, but also about how poultry is still as safe as it has always been, and a very popular main course for many meals. And happy Thanksgiving to you and everyone else here, and if the gentleman from North Carolina would come and take the Chair as the chairman of the Livestock Subcommittee, I would now recognize the gentleman from California, Mr. Costa.

Mr. LARSEN. Mr. Chairman.

The CHAIRMAN. Yes.

Mr. LARSEN. Was than an invitation?

The CHAIRMAN. Yes, you come down and we will take good care of you.

Mr. LARSEN. Thank you.

Mr. COSTA. Hope you have a lot of turkey, Mr. Chairman. Thank you, Mr. Chairman, and the ranking member, for holding this hearing today. I think it is very timely and it is appropriate.

I have several questions, Dr. DeHaven, and I appreciate your appropriate responses. The U.N.'s Food and Agriculture Organization has pledged $150 million to deal with it on an international basis, and you have talked about the $18 million that is in the President's proposal. Out of the $150 million that has been pledged, I understand there is actually $25 million that they have available. Is that part of the $18 million that you spoke of?

Dr. DeHAVEN. No, that is separate funding coming through the FAO. The President's request for emergency funding has——

Mr. COSTA. Above and beyond the $18 million?

Dr. DeHAVEN. Above and beyond those monies.

Mr. COSTA. How would you describe the efforts? We are obviously almost daily reading in the news outlets about what is going on in China and other parts of Southeast Asia and in Europe to deal with the various strains. Could you give us a brief descriptive as to how you believe that our foreign partners are doing in terms of with the various strains in combating this animal disease?

Dr. DeHAVEN. I think the response to this particular virus is as varied as there are numbers of countries that have been affected. Some of the affected countries have a good infrastructure in place, have a good commercial industry already willing and able to assist with the overall effort. And then at the opposite extreme, we have individual farmers, producers who have smaller flocks——

Mr. COSTA. I understand when they are running wild in the villages and those kinds of circumstances it is much more difficult. Where would you say from the international perspective is the greatest problematic area that we should be concerned about?

Dr. DeHAVEN. Contrary to the statement by the chairman, I have not yet traveled to Southeast Asia. I will be there beginning December 9, and that is the kind of information I hope to gather firsthand.

Having heard from the delegation that accompanied Secretary Leavitt in his Southeast Asia tour a number of weeks ago, I am hearing some countries, such as Laos, just simply do not have the infrastructure. And what they need is not only the technical expertise on how to effectively deal with the virus, given their particular situation, but also assistance in procuring vaccination, training vaccination crews, training culling crews, everything that would be necessary that we take for granted that we have in place here.

Mr. COSTA. After your visit, Doctor, it just seems to me it would be appropriate if you were to get back to the committee and Members of Congress with the Department of Health and Human Services. If we are going to try to avoid a pandemic situation here, it seems to me, to use your terminology, we are going to have to triage this. And the best way to deal with triaging a situation that is international in scope is to figure out where the problematic areas are and, hopefully, try to concentrate our resources in those areas where we think they can do the most good.

Getting a handle on that sooner rather than later, I think, is going to be critical to avoiding any potential of a pandemic situation.

Dr. DeHaven. I very much appreciate that comment, and that is precisely the purpose of my visit, is to get a handle on what is the situation in individual countries and how can we, working through organizations like the FAO and the OIE, how can we best provide the assistance that is going to best attack the virus given the situation in the individual countries.

Mr. Costa. Last question. I would like to get a little more clarity. As you described the stockpiling of the various vaccines to deal with combating the spread of it within the animals, it is not clear to me when we are talking about our supply of vaccine where that difference lies between vaccines for humans. Could you add a little more information? Where is our stockpiling with regard to the need for people?

Dr. DeHaven. My comments, Congressman, were directed strictly at stockpiling of vaccine for use in poultry.

Mr. Costa. Right, that is what I understood.

Dr. DeHaven. So we have 40 million in doses in the bank, 30 million we will be ordering, and with the President's request, if approved, the ability to purchase 40 million more doses of vaccine. Again, all directed specifically at the virus for use in poultry.

There is a concerted effort on the public health side to develop a human vaccine and to stockpile that. I would simply have to defer to my public health colleagues to give you a status report on where they are in developing and producing that vaccine.

Mr. Costa. One quick follow-up, Mr. Chairman. On the coordination effort, as you mentioned in your comments earlier, in California we have an active poultry program. How would you describe the coordination on a State-Federal relationship with the various agricultural departments throughout the country?

Dr. DeHaven. First of all, let me say that you have just got an outstanding poultry industry in the State of California. We got to know——

Mr. Costa. We think so. Thank you.

Dr. DeHaven. We got to know them firsthand. And heaven forbid we have another outbreak of poultry disease, but if we do, I hope we have the kind of cooperation and energy that we had in California in dealing with exotic Newcastle disease, both in terms of the State agency that we dealt with, California Department of Food and Agriculture, as well as the poultry industry. The cooperation was tremendous and resulted in our success.

In APHIS, we are very, very proud of our accomplishments, and many of those accomplishments go to a number of successful seiz-eradication efforts. But I am always quick to add that everything we accomplish in that regard is done in concert with State departments of agriculture. All of our programs are cooperative in nature. So when we say that we have a program, whether it is for avian influenza or brucellosis eradication, we have a program in cooperation with the State agencies.

So all of our efforts would be done in concert, and I feel comfortable in saying that we have a good working relationship, State and Federal, in all 50 States. And indeed our emergency response mechanism is based upon a joint State-Federal response where the State veterinarian and our Federal veterinarian would be codirectors of that effort. So we emphasize that.

We have in place area emergency coordinators whose full-time job is emergency response coordination, and much of what they do is coordinate with the State agencies that would be part of that response. So I feel comfortable in saying that that is in place.

Mr. COSTA. Thank you very much, Mr. Chairman.

Mr. HAYES [presiding]. The gentleman from Tennessee, Mr. Davis.

Mr. DAVIS. Mr. Chairman and ranking member, I deeply appreciate the opportunity today to discuss with Dr. DeHaven the possibility of an outbreak of flu and how we can contain it. Since Hurricane Katrina struck the Gulf Coast this past August, there has been a lot of media scrutiny over the government's ability to respond to the disasters that affect large populations and land areas. The question has been asked more than once will the government be able to respond to lethal pandemics, like the bird flu, if we were to have an outbreak in the United States?

While I certainly think many in the media are guilty of using fear tactics in order to drive up their viewership, I do think it is a valid question. Is the United States, the most advanced, richest country in the world, prepared to handle an outbreak of the fast spreading lethal disease that can mutate quickly? I hope that is the case. I think that is a problem for many of us if we are not.

It seems every day we hear more about the bird flu. We hear about the different strains. We hear it is killing people and spreading rather quickly around the globe. As a matter of fact, we have had three outbreaks here. And I think it is a compliment to the USDA and to our health department that we were able to contain that.

I represent a district that has a large area of poultry producers. As a youngster growing up, we raised broilers on our farm. And in the area of the Cumberland Mountains, the Cumberland Plateau, which I represent, there are several different companies that today are involved in poultry production, mainly for fryers. And it is important, I think, that we realize this is something as a major exporter and as a major producer of poultry that we have to contain.

I remember 20 years ago Human Immunodeficiency Virus, HIV, coming to the forefront. I also remember another term, Acquired Immune Deficiency Syndrome, or AIDS. So we went through a period of time then and currently trying to find a cure. We still have this virus around. This flu virus, the avian flu virus, will probably be around for many years to come. We have found a way not necessarily to contain but at least to prevent.

So my concern is what is USDA doing in areas where there is high poultry production like in the district I represent in Tennessee, what are we doing to tell the farmers what signs to look for; and if there are indications of developing the bird flu, how can they contain that? And if there is an outbreak, how will they be able to actually identify it?

It is my hope that USDA, through their agencies in the rural areas, are at least getting an information flow to alert of the symptoms and alert as to preventive ways to keep bird flu from occurring in their flocks. Are you doing that?

Dr. DEHAVEN. Indeed, we are. Let me first address, Mr. Davis, if I could, our response mechanisms. I just mentioned that we have in place at the State level a State-Federal cooperative emergency response capability at the State level with the ability to supplement that State level response regionally from similar organizations in other States in the country. So we have that ability to add blocks, if you will, to a State-level response, and then have the ability to coordinate multistate response regionally and then nationally.

We have been responding, as you indicated, to outbreaks of avian influenza for decades and have experience. What we do is prepare for and respond to those kinds of situations. We do have a unique situation with this particular virus, in that it has shown the ability to produce significant disease in humans, and that would present some unique challenges to us as we work to eliminate that particular virus while also protecting our people who might be involved in the response to that mechanism. And, indeed, we have appropriate protocols in place to provide for that kind of protection.

In terms of what are we telling producers, I would go back to our Biosecurity for the Birds Campaign, a $4.4 million campaign if I am not mistaken, that we instituted a couple of years ago. It is aimed at the individual producer and what can they do on a day-to-day basis to keep unwanted pathogens off the farm and out of the poultry house.

Part of that outreach campaign is if you see unusual mortality, decrease in egg production for laying flocks or anything like that, to report those to State authorities so we can quickly respond. We emphasize the fact that the key to eradication of an incursion is early detection and rapid response.

So we have the rapid response mechanisms in place. Early detection would rely upon participation and cooperation of the industry. Here again, I would emphasize the tremendous cooperation and relationship that we have with the industry both at the national level with the National Turkey Federation, the Chicken Council, and other organizations, but also at the State level. Virtually every poultry producing State has a State poultry organization where we have those contacts at the State level.

Indeed, it was working with the Virginia Poultry Federation with the low-path outbreak in 2002 and 2003 that largely contributed to our successful effort there. If we were to have a huge multistate outbreak, we do have now the capability to call upon the resources of the entire Federal Government.

FEMA recently identified an emergency support function specific for food, agriculture, and water, and APHIS is one of the lead agencies; meaning that if we were to have a large agricultural emergency, just like FEMA can call upon resources of the entire government to respond to a hurricane, we would have at our disposal all of the resources of the government under this emergency support function for food, agriculture, and water.

Mr. DAVIS. Thank you, Dr. DeHaven. I yield back the remainder of my time.

Mr. HAYES. Mr. Etheridge.

Mr. ETHERIDGE. Thank you. Dr. DeHaven, thank you for being here.

You spoke of significant funding increases and the administration's plan to combat avian flu, and as you have mentioned we have been battling it in spots, Virginia being one of the places several years ago which impacted our ability to ship product. My own State of North Carolina has a significant population. It is well over a billion dollar industry in North Carolina.

Specifically, though, you mentioned an increase of roughly 40 million additional doses being added to the existing USDA animal vaccine bank for avian flu. I do not know if I missed this in your testimony or not, but what is the approximate number of doses available right now in USDA's vaccine bank?

That is an important piece as we talk about the concerns, and I think we can allay the fears of a lot of people if we had some idea of what kind of numbers we are talking about.

Dr. DeHaven. Let me answer your question in just a second, and point out that vaccination would be typically not our first means of response.

Mr. Etheridge. I understand that. But it is important as a broader context.

Dr. DeHaven. Indeed.

Mr. Etheridge. If it becomes a multistate piece, as you just mentioned.

Dr. DeHaven. We have in our vaccine bank right now 40 million doses, we are contracting to purchase an additional 30 million doses, and if the President's request is approved, we would contract for an additional 40 million.

I should clarify, however, of the 40 million we currently have in the bank, 20 million is for an H5 subtype. It has been tested and shown effective against this particular virus. The remaining 20 million doses are for H7, and presumably would not be effective against this particular Southeast Asian H5N1.

Mr. Etheridge. So, in effect, we have 20 million doses?

Dr. DeHaven. Correct.

Mr. Etheridge. Now, if you put that in perspective to what we are talking about in terms of the magnitude of the number of birds out there, poultry, it is not a very large bank.

Dr. DeHaven. It is in fact a relatively small percentage of the total poultry population. But even if we did choose to use vaccination, it would be typically on a limited basis to vaccinate to contain an area where there was infection. Ring vaccination, if you will.

Mr. Etheridge. Sure. I think it is important to have that and know where we are headed, because poultry is a huge part, it is a substantial part of the economic stream in rural America, and certainly is important to our export markets around the world.

Dr. DeHaven. Indeed. And to have all contingencies available to us is precisely why we are seeking to add to that vaccine bank.

Mr. Etheridge. Let me follow that up, because due to the large number of animal populations in our State, which really goes beyond poultry, and if you remember several years ago when hoof and mouth disease became a big issue with the outbreak in Europe, a number of tabletop exercises took place in the States, one of which was in my home State, and I think you got a lot of people's attention to see how quickly that could spread all across America. USDA was involved and all the agencies you have mentioned already.

As a result of that, obviously the quarantine that would have had to have been put in place if you had that kind of outbreak would not only have affected animals but would have affected the ability of populations to move, and would have had a real impact on our economic stream. So that leads to the question, because it affects roads, it affects travel, its affects transportation, so it wasn't a very pretty view when we started to look at it, can you tell us what USDA would do in the immediate aftermath should the avian flu become an outbreak?

Because I think it is important for this committee to know that there is a plan in place at the State, Federal and local level. And hopefully someone has been out there doing a test on it. What would you do if we had a major outbreak someplace in the country? I know we have had isolated places, but give us some assurance of what you would do in that case if, number one, we found it in wild birds, and, secondly, if it were discovered on a number of farms in a geographic area somewhere in this country, North Carolina, Virginia, or wherever.

Dr. DeHaven. As I mentioned, part of the monies would go towards wild bird surveillance for precisely what you are talking about, and we would look at wild birds and the surveillance of wild birds as an early warning sign. If we in fact find a highly pathogen virus, whether it is the Southeast Asia virus or another high-path virus, we in effect have an early warning that, hey, the virus is close. And while we have been diligent, all the more reason to be extremely vigilant in areas where we have found the virus in wild birds.

There is absolutely no way to control wild bird populations. We cannot eradicate wild migratory birds, but they could provide a very effective early warning system. If we have a report of an unusual situation, higher mortality than normal in a production flock, for example, we have a cadre of 450 veterinarians across the country trained in foreign animal disease diagnosis. Our goal is to have one of those people on that farm within 4 hours. We would have samples submitted and presumably preliminary lab results in 12 to 24 hours after that. And if it were confirmed positive, we would activate our incident command system immediately and gather those people on site.

One of the first things that would happen, even if we had a highly suspicious situation that was not yet confirmed, we would discuss with the State authorities the relative benefit of imposing a State quarantine on that premise until we had a confirmed diagnosis.

But initially we would impose State quarantine. We have the ability to impose Federal quarantines very quickly, if need be, where the State quarantine can restrict intrastate movement and the Federal quarantine can also restrict interstate movement.

So the first thing is to contain it where it is. Of the known positive flocks, wc would quickly depopulate those as we did a couple of things. One, start surveillance testing in that area, which would be presumably also under quarantine. So we would do surveillance testing, but we would also be doing some epidemiological studies to find out what movements had come on to that premise, what movement had gone off of that particular premise, as to where it might have spread and then follow up from there.

Mr. ETHERIDGE. Possibly to other farmers.

Dr. DEHAVEN. Correct.

Mr. ETHERIDGE. Let me just interrupt, because I know my time is running out. North Carolina has an excellent program. We have a great State veterinarian. The State General Assembly has given substantial authority to him to work at the State level, of course, and working with USDA. But certainly if something, a major outbreak would come, it is going to take all the resources of everyone working together.

Dr. DEHAVEN. And, indeed, the State animal health response mechanism in North Carolina is a model program. It is outstanding.

Mr. ETHERIDGE. Thank you. Thank you, Mr. Chairman. I yield back.

Mr. HAYES. Dr. DeHaven, our duck hunter has left, but I am still here. Is there anything that someone, a hunter, for example, if noticing something should turn it into their local USDA office or Wildlife Commission, anything to add there?

Dr. DEHAVEN. Either to the State Wildlife Agency or to the State Department of Agriculture. Anything like that they should notify those officials and get that bird to a State laboratory for diagnostic testing. Virtually any of the State laboratories can do that testing or can get samples to the Federal laboratory where we can do the testing, and I think that would be a prudent thing to do. But at the same time, in the interest of not causing undue alarm, there has been a lot of testing going on and at this point there is absolutely no evidence to suggest that we have high-path avian influenza in wild birds, commercial birds, or for that matter humans in the United States. But, again, appropriate to be vigilant.

Mr. HAYES. Dr. DeHaven, as usual, you have been very concise, very professional, very thorough, and very reassuring. I think it is important to have this information available. In that context you have spoken very well for sound science today.

Is there anything you would like to add that would assist people in understanding and being comfortable with how you and the Department are handling this, many of the things they might do?

Dr. DEHAVEN. Mr. Chairman, thank you for this opportunity, as well as the opportunity to summarize.

I think that the President has laid out a very good strategy where, on the public health side, we would prepare for a potential for this virus to mutate and become a pandemic-type virus, and prepare by developing and stockpiling a vaccine and stockpiling antiviral medications.

But the President's strategy also includes monies for us to attack the virus at its source. The potential for a pandemic is greatly reduced if we can assist affected countries and reduce the virus load and thereby reduce or eliminate the potential for this to become a pandemic virus.

And the President's plan also includes additional monies for us to have increased vigilance, surveillance, testing capacity, and outreach to our industry domestically should we have an incursion. We have been preparing in APHIS for 20 years for avian influenza outbreaks. We have responded successfully to eradicate avian influenza on a number of occasions, and we have appropriately increased our level of vigilance because of the virus that is in Southeast Asia.

But, again, I would emphasize that while we are vigilant, we have the mechanisms for response in place on the animal side, there is no evidence to suggest that we have that H5N1 virus either in animals or in people in the United States. So as the chairman indicated, he will be enjoying Thanksgiving turkey, as will the DeHaven family. We will likewise be having turkey for Thanksgiving and enjoying it very much.

Thank you.

Mr. HAYES. Thank you, sir, and that is my plan as well. I might only add that having seen the demonstration that I am sure you have seen, given satellite imagery and Global Positioning System technology, the Department and the States have the ability to quickly identify and graphically display the actual geographic areas should there be an outbreak that needs to be quarantined or dealt with.

So that is another piece of the puzzle, that, again, given technology and modern day methods that provide us additional preventive measures in case something should happen. So again thank you very much, and we do look forward to turkey day.

Without objection, today's hearing will remain open for 10 days to receive additional material and supplemental written responses from witnesses to any question posed by a member of the panel.

Having said that, the hearing of the House Committee on Agriculture is adjourned. Thank you very much, Doctor.

[Whereupon, at 11:48 a.m., the committee was adjourned.]

[Material submitted for inclusion in the record follows:]

STATEMENT OF RON DEHAVEN

Mr. Chairman and members of the committee, thank you for the opportunity to testify regarding the Department of Agriculture's extensive efforts to protect U.S. poultry from avian influenza. Our efforts over the years, in cooperation with many Federal, State, and industry partners, have been highly successful in preventing serious incursions of this disease from abroad and, when necessary, taking swift action to control and eradicate discoveries in the United States.

As has been reported, H5N1, a highly pathogenic strain of avian influenza, has been spreading across poultry populations in several Southeast Asian countries, Russia and eastern European countries in recent months. There have also been documented cases of the virus affecting humans who have been in direct contact with sick birds. There is worldwide concern that the H5N1 virus might mutate, cross the species barrier and touch off a human influenza pandemic.

With this in mind, USDA's poultry health safeguarding programs are more important than ever. These programs are based on preventative regulatory and anti-smuggling measures designed to mitigate the risk of the virus entering the United States; targeted, aggressive disease surveillance in domestic poultry; and emergency response capabilities that ensure coordinated action with our partners in the event of detection. We take these responsibilities very seriously, and have bolstered all the components of our safeguarding program in response to the evolving avian influenza situation overseas.

We also believe it is critical to effectively address the disease in the poultry population in Southeast Asia. Implementation of effective biosecurity measures and control and eradication programs will go a long way toward reducing the amount of virus in these H5N1-affected countries and minimize the potential for the virus to spread to poultry in other areas of the world. These actions, if effectively implemented, would diminish the potential for a human influenza pandemic.

I will soon travel extensively in Southeast Asia in an effort to evaluate the animal health infrastructure in Southeast Asia and determine what steps can be taken to improve disease safeguarding and surveillance programs in the region. I know that there is widespread concern in Asia regarding avian influenza, as well as a strong commitment to working with the international community to address the disease and improve the animal health infrastructure in countries like Vietnam, Cambodia, Laos, Indonesia and Thailand. This is why it is imperative that the United States remains engaged and share resources and expertise with officials in these countries. I have also just returned from a United

Nations World Health Organization meeting on avian influenza in Geneva, Switzerland. It is clear this is an international effort.

Now let me turn to preparedness efforts here in the United States. The National Strategy for Pandemic Influenza, announced by President Bush on November 1, reflects the importance of these proactive measures on the animal health front. The President requested $91.35 million in emergency funding for USDA to further intensify its surveillance here at home and to deliver increased assistance to countries impacted by the disease, in hopes of preventing further spread of avian influenza.

On the international front, $18.35 million of the emergency funding for USDA is needed for additional bisosecurity, surveillance, and diagnostic measures. This funding would significantly advance USDA's efforts that build on the Food and Agriculture Organization's work to prevent, control and eradicate avian influenza where it currently exists in Asia.

To continue strengthening our domestic activities, $73 million of the USDA emergency funding is needed for stockpiling animal vaccine, surveillance and diagnostics, anti-smuggling and investigative efforts, research and development, planning and preparedness and staffing and management. The objective of all these efforts will be to prevent, control and eradicate any future findings of the H5 and H7 strains of avian influenza in the U.S. commercial broiler and live bird marketing system.

This is just a brief overview of what is an important request to Congress by the Administration. We appreciate your support of our efforts and look forward to working with the Congress as it considers the President's emergency funding request for pandemic influenza.

Now, I would like to turn to information on avian influenza necessary for our discussion regarding the disease, its potential effects on poultry in the United States, the steps USDA is taking to look for the disease and prepare for any detection, trade related matters, and some important food safety information of which we should always be aware.

Background on Avian Influenza

Avian influenza viruses are actually in the same family of viruses that cause flu in people every year. There is a flu season every year in birds, just as there is a flu season for humans. And as you would expect, some forms of avian influenza are more severe than others.

Avian influenza viruses can infect chickens, turkeys, pheasants, quail, ducks, geese, and guinea fowl as well as other varieties of birds, including migratory waterfowl. Transmission of the virus from one bird to another occurs through direct contact typically through contact with respiratory secretions or feces.

Worldwide, there are many strains of the avian influenza virus, which again can cause varying degrees of illness in poultry. These viruses are characterized by two different proteins on the surface of the virus. One is called hemaglutinin, or H for short, and the other one is a neuraminidase protein, or N for short. There are 16 known H proteins and 9 known N proteins, for a possible combination of 144 different characterizations of virus.

With regard to birds, avian influenza viruses are further divided into two groups low pathogenic avian influenza, or low path, and highly pathogenic, or high path, viruses.

Pathogenesis refers to the ability of the virus to produce disease, with the highly pathogenic viruses producing far more severe clinical signs and higher mortality in birds than you would expect with the low pathogenic avian influenza virus.

Low pathogenic avian influenza has been identified in the United States and around the world since the early 1900's. It is relatively common to detect low pathogenic, just as human flu viruses are a common finding in people. However, most avian influenza viruses found in birds do not pose any significant health risk to humans.

Highly pathogenic avian influenza (HPAI) has been found in poultry in the United States three times: 1924, 1983 and 2004. The 1983 outbreak was the largest, ultimately resulting in the destruction of 17 million birds in Pennsylvania and Virginia before that virus was finally contained and eradicated. By contrast, an isolated HPAI incident in a flock of 6,600 birds in Texas was quickly found and eradicated in 2004. There were no reports of human health problems in connection with any of those outbreaks.

In domestic poultry, the greatest concern has been infections with H5 or H7 strains, which are either highly pathogenic or low pathogenic avian influenza. The low pathogenic H5 and H7 viruses are always of a concern because of their potential to mutate to the highly pathogenic version of the disease.

Again, speaking strictly with regard to birds, only H5 and H7 subtypes of the avian influenza viruses have ever been shown to be highly pathogenic. The most recent outbreaks in the United States that I just mentioned both happened to be H5N2 viruses. The virus that is currently circulating in Asia is an H5N1 virus.

As I mentioned earlier, this particular H5N1 virus is also unique in that it has been transmitted from birds to humans, most of who had reported extensive direct contact with infected birds. I think it is important to emphasize, however, that there is no evidence at this time that the H5N1 virus that is currently circulating in Asia is in the United States, either in birds or humans.

Safeguarding Efforts

The Federal Government is actively engaged in the global effort to help eradicate highly pathogenic avian influenza (HPAI). The primary goal of this effort is to minimize any potential threat to human or animal health. USDA has been working closely with the U.S. Agency for International Development (USAID) to support animal health intervention in infected countries to establish safer, science-based agricultural practices in order to meet internationally accepted animal health standards and to facilitate trade.

Safer agricultural practices can result in greater food safety, food security, and public health improvement. By helping these countries prepare for, manage, or eradicate outbreaks, USDA can reduce the risk of high pathogenic avian influenza or other animal diseases spreading to the United States.

USDA is also engaged in an interagency working group with the Department of Interior that will use modeling to evaluate the role of wildlife in foreign animal disease threats. The initial diseases of focus will be foot and mouth disease and avian influenza.

Furthermore, USDA and other Federal agencies are communicating and collaborating with Federal public health agencies, including the Centers for Disease Control (CDC) in the Department of Health and Human Services, regarding avian influenza prevention, preparedness, and response activities and programs. Avian influenza demonstrates the need for increasing the links between animal and human health agencies, domestically and internationally, to respond to emerging infectious diseases at the animal/human interface.

There are other important efforts USDA has employed to keep the H5N1 virus and others out of the United States. As a primary safeguard, the Department's Animal and Plant Health Inspection Service (APHIS) maintains trade restrictions on the importation of live poultry, birds and unprocessed poultry products from all affected countries. Heat-treated poultry meat and eggs from countries with high pathogenic avian influenza (HPAI) are considered eligible for importation from countries with equivalent meat inspection systems. Imports of live birds, poultry and unprocessed poultry products, may resume after APHIS has completed a regionalization analysis that identifies the entire country or zone within the affected-country as disease-free.

APHIS' Smuggling, Interdiction, and Trade Compliance teams, as well as our colleagues with the Department of Homeland Security's Customs and Border Protection, have been alerted and are vigilantly on the lookout for any poultry or poultry products that might be smuggled into the United States from any of the affected countries.

Additionally, USDA quarantines and tests imported live birds from countries not known to have cases of infection to make sure that pet birds and other fowl do not inadvertently introduce disease into the United States.

We also have an ongoing surveillance program that targets avian influenza and other serious diseases in commercial flocks. The idea of surveillance is simply that if avian influenza is here, we want to find it very quickly and then respond to eliminate it. Early detection and rapid response are the keys to minimize the impact on our poultry production as well as minimize any impact with regard to trade restrictions.

APHIS conducts more than one million tests a year for avian influenza. USDA's Agricultural Research Service developed—and APHIS validated—a rapid test for avian influenza that has proven highly effective in screening for the disease. The test has been distributed to National Animal Health Laboratory Network labs all across the country.

The rapid test also supports our targeted surveillance efforts at live bird markets in the northeastern United States. USDA has also been working closely with the State Agricultural Departments and industry representatives to increase surveillance at these markets in recent years. This cooperative program is designed to prevent, diagnose and, if found, eliminate any of the H5 or H7 subtypes of virus in those markets.

I would be remiss if I did not mention the outstanding support of the U.S. commercial poultry industry in terms of producers' vigilance in applying and adhering to good biosecurity practices on the farm. Biosecurity simply means applying some very practical, common sense measures to keep from bringing unwanted germs onto the farm or into the poultry houses.

I also want to emphasize that for the last several years APHIS has conducted a major outreach campaign called "Biosecurity for the Birds." The campaign places informational materials directly into the hands of commercial poultry producers, as well as those raising poultry in their backyards. All of the brochures and fact sheets are available in several languages and emphasize the need for good biosecurity and disease surveillance programs to reduce the possibility of bringing any disease, not just avian influenza, on the farm or into their back yard.

The Department of the Interior is responsible for managing wildlife, including migratory birds under various laws such as the Migratory Bird Treaty Act, and for ensuring public health on the more than 500 million acres of land that it manages across the country. To carry out these responsibilities, biologists within the Department of Interior's Fish and Wildlife Service and U.S. Geological Survey have been strategically sampling migratory birds for H5N1 in the Pacific Flyway.

These efforts complement a series of ongoing avian influenza studies being conducted by USDA's Agricultural Research Service (ARS) and its university partners in Alaska where birds that regularly migrate between Asia and North America are known to congregate. The ARS seven-year collaboration with the University of Alaska has evaluated over 12,000 Alaskan samples and to date has found no evidence of high pathogenic avian influenza virus.

APHIS' Wildlife Services (WS) has also provided assistance to minimize threats to the public and animal health through its National Wildlife Disease Surveillance and Emergency Response Plan. Recently, WS has worked closely with Texas, North Carolina, New Jersey, Arizona and Nevada to conduct sampling of waterfowl, geese, and exotic birds for avian influenza.

EMERGENCY RESPONSE

USDA has in place a robust emergency response program designed to complement our surveillance efforts. When we have unexpected poultry, or for that matter livestock, illnesses or deaths on a farm, we immediately conduct a foreign animal disease investigation. We have a cadre of specially trained veterinarians who can be on site within four hours to conduct an initial examination and submit samples for laboratory testing.

As the Committee knows, APHIS is not new to disease incursions and successful eradication efforts. In conjunction with our State colleagues, there are State-level emergency response teams on standby. These teams will typically be on site within 24 hours of a presumptive diagnosis of avian influenza or any other significant foreign animal disease. Destruction of the affected flocks would be our primary concern and course of action. We would also likely immediately work with State or tribes to impose State-level quarantines and movement restrictions.

For highly pathogenic avian influenza as well as for low pathogenic H5 and H7 subtypes, APHIS would work with States to quarantine affected premises and clean and disinfect those premises after the birds have been depopulated and disposed. All positive HPNAI flocks would be depopulated and meat from affected flocks would not enter the animal or human food chain. Surveillance testing would also be conducted in the quarantine zone and surrounding area to ensure that the virus has been completely eradicated. An essential part of a successful emergency response program is effective communication with the media and the public. This is especially important given the concern right now regarding avian influenza and potential risks to human health. To be prepared in the event of a detection—whether it be high pathogenic or low pathogenic avian influenza—USDA has been coordinating with its counterparts at other Federal agencies, State Agriculture Departments, and industry organizations to ensure consistent messages regarding the strain of the disease found, the steps being taken in response, and the potential effects to poultry and, if appropriate, human health. In fact, USDA will be participating in a government-wide tabletop exercise with a focus on avian influenza. Coordination will be vital to our ability to deliver important information, while maintaining public confidence in, among other things, the food supply and public health system.

USDA also maintains a bank of avian influenza vaccines for animals in the event that the vaccine would be a preferred course of action in any outbreak situation. I need to stress here, however, that wide-scale vaccination of poultry is not an effective safeguard against avian influenza. Rather, animal vaccination could be used in response to a detection of the disease in the United States to create barriers against further spread and assist with our overall control and eradication measures.

Funding included in the emergency request would augment the current animal vaccine bank by an additional 40 million doses. This expansion to the animal vaccine bank would be critical in the event of a large-scale avian influenza situation in the United States.

TRADE ISSUES

As we know, outbreaks of significant foreign animal diseases are extremely costly in terms of domestic control and eradication efforts. However, we have seen that lost export markets can be even more damaging to the U.S. economy. As part of its planning to address avian influenza, then, APHIS has taken a lead role in facilitating international consideration of new trade standards for AI. For example, USDA actively supported the drafting of an improved World Animal Health (OIE) standard for avian influenza adopted in May 2005. Under the recently amended OIE guidelines, OIE members are obligated to report any positive NAI—or Notifiable Avian Influenza (NAI) test result. This includes the reporting of all highly pathogenic strains of AI, as well as the H5 and H7 subtypes of low pathogenic AI detected in commercial poultry flocks.

Notifiable avian influenza-related trade restrictions on poultry products should be limited to the affected "zone", e.g. country, state, region, or "compartment," e.g. isolating commercial poultry from migratory waterfowl or wildlife. The OIE does not recommend trade restrictions for non-H5 or H7 low pathogenic subtypes.

Properly cooked meat and pasteurized egg products are considered safe-to-trade products and are safe for human consumption. Since heat has shown to destroy the virus, the OIE recently proposed draft guidelines for inactivating the virus using heat-treatments.

APHIS continues to work with its trading partners to promote the application of the new OIE standard. As just one case in point, intensive negotiations resulted in Mexico's recent agreement to lift all remaining import restrictions on States that have reported cases of low pathogenic avian influenza in recent years.

The detection of high pathogenic avian influenza in Texas in 2004 led to the closure of several export markets to U.S. poultry and poultry products. However, in that case APHIS worked to not only control and eradicate the disease, but to demonstrate to trading partners that the measures put in place were effective in controlling and eradicating the virus. APHIS urged trading partners to regionalize the United States for the disease, effectively allowing trade in poultry and products to continue from unaffected areas. These efforts were successful in reopening export markets.

Under prevailing international trade agreements, U.S. trading partners are obligated to consider a regionalization request from USDA, and countries must base their decisions on sound, demonstrable scientific grounds. The United States would certainly do this in response to a regionalization request from another country, and we expect—and will hold—other countries to this same standard should high pathogenic avian influenza be detected again in this country.

FOOD SAFETY

If high pathogenic avian influenza were to be detected in the United States, I want to emphasize that the U.S. surveillance system would find the disease, and our emergency response system would quickly contain the outbreak while eradication efforts begin. The chance that infected poultry would ever enter the human food chain would be extremely low. That is in part because we have inspection personnel from USDA's Food Safety and Inspection Service assigned to every federally inspected meat, poultry and egg product plant in the United States. Poultry products for public consumption are inspected for signs of disease both before and after slaughter. The "inspected for wholesomeness by the U.S. Department of Agriculture" seal ensures that this poultry is free from visible signs of disease.

No human cases of avian influenza have been confirmed from eating properly prepared poultry. In addition to proper processing in the plants, proper handling and cooking of poultry provides protection from viruses and bacteria including avian influenza.

I want to reiterate that proper food safety practices are important every day. USDA reminds consumers each day—and especially as we look ahead to Thanksgiving—that there are basic food safety steps to follow. It applies to any raw meat, poultry, or fish. That is clean, separate, cook, and chill.

By clean we mean always wash your hands with warm water and soap for at least 20 seconds. After cutting raw meats, wash cutting board, knife, and counter tops with hot, soapy water. By separate we mean do not cross-contaminate. Keep raw meat, poultry, fish and their juices away from other foods.

Cooking the meat and poultry to the proper temperatures using a food thermometer is the only sure way to know that you have cooked that product properly. A high enough temperature will destroy bacteria and viruses in poultry products. USDA specifically recommends cooking ground turkey and chicken to a temperature of 165 degrees Fahrenheit; cook chicken and turkey breasts to 170 degrees Fahrenheit; and whole birds, legs, thighs and wings to 180 degrees Fahrenheit. Obviously, never consume raw or undercooked poultry or poultry products.

And then chill meat products promptly after serving in the refrigerator. Always refrigerate perishable foods within 2 hours of taking it out of the refrigerator or having prepared it by proper cooking. Whole roasts, hams, and turkeys should be sliced or cut into smaller pieces or portions before storing them in the refrigerator or freezer. Turkey legs, wings, and thighs may be left whole. Refrigerate or freeze leftovers in shallow containers. Wrap or cover the food. And as a reminder, refrigerators should be at 40 degrees Fahrenheit or lower, and freezers should be at 0 degrees Fahrenheit or lower.

You should also use cooked leftovers after Thanksgiving within 3 to 4 days to be safe.

Consumers with questions about the safe storage, handling, or preparation of meat, poultry, and egg products can contact the USDA Meat and Poultry Hotline at (800) MP-Hotline, that is (800) 674–6854. The hotline is available in English and Spanish and can be reached from 10:00 a.m. to 4:00 p.m. Eastern Standard Time, Monday through Friday. Consumers may also check out our Web site at *www.fsis.usda.gov* to ask our virtual representative questions 24 hours a day.

Mr. Chairman and members of the committee, thank you again for holding this hearing and allowing me to provide this important overview regarding avian influenza. I have covered a lot of ground in my remarks and will be happy to answer your questions.

○